Name	
Address	
Phone No.	
Mobile No.	
Email	
Emergency Information	
Notes	

MEDICAL HISTORY

Date Of Birth	
Blood Type	
Chronic Conditions	
Food Allergies	
Medical Allergies	
Maintenance Medication	
Physician	
Notes	

Immunizations

Date	Vaccinations	Hospital/Clinic	Notes

MEDICAL CONTACTS

Name	
Type	
Hospital / Clinic	
Phone No.	
Mobile No.	
Email	
Notes	

Name	
Type	
Hospital / Clinic	
Phone No.	
Mobile No.	
Email	
Notes	

Name	
Type	
Hospital / Clinic	
Phone No.	
Mobile No.	
Email	
Notes	

MEDICAL CONTACTS

Name	
Type	
Hospital / Clinic	
Phone No.	
Mobile No.	
Email	
Notes	

Name	
Type	
Hospital / Clinic	
Phone No.	
Mobile No.	
Email	
Notes	

Name	
Type	
Hospital / Clinic	
Phone No.	
Mobile No.	
Email	
Notes	

Doctor Visit Log

Date		Time:
Doctor		
Hospital / Clinic		
Phone No.		

Reasons For The Visit	Questions To Ask
Symptoms	Prescription / Tests

Pain Scale	1	2	3	4	5

Next Appointment :

Follow Up Notes:

Doctor Visit Log

Date		Time:
Doctor		
Hospital / Clinic		
Phone No.		

Reasons For The Visit	Questions To Ask
Symptoms	**Prescription / Tests**

Pain Scale	1	2	3	4	5

Next Appointment :

Follow Up Notes:

Doctor Visit Log

Date		Time:
Doctor		
Hospital / Clinic		
Phone No.		

Reasons For The Visit	Questions To Ask
Symptoms	Prescription / Tests

Pain Scale	1	2	3	4	5

Next Appointment :

Follow Up Notes:

Doctor Visit Log

Date		Time:
Doctor		
Hospital / Clinic		
Phone No.		

Reasons For The Visit	Questions To Ask
Symptoms	Prescription / Tests

Pain Scale	1	2	3	4	5

Next Appointment :

Follow Up Notes:

Doctor Visit Log

Date		Time:
Doctor		
Hospital / Clinic		
Phone No.		

Reasons For The Visit	Questions To Ask
Symptoms	**Prescription / Tests**

Pain Scale	1	2	3	4	5

Next Appointment :

Follow Up Notes:

Doctor Visit Log

Date		Time:
Doctor		
Hospital / Clinic		
Phone No.		

Reasons For The Visit	Questions To Ask

Symptoms	Prescription / Tests

Pain Scale	1	2	3	4	5

Next Appointment :

Follow Up Notes:

Doctor Visit Log

Date		Time:
Doctor		
Hospital / Clinic		
Phone No.		

Reasons For The Visit	Questions To Ask
Symptoms	Prescription / Tests

Pain Scale	1	2	3	4	5

Next Appointment :

Follow Up Notes:

Doctor Visit Log

Date		Time:
Doctor		
Hospital / Clinic		
Phone No.		

Reasons For The Visit	Questions To Ask
Symptoms	Prescription / Tests

Pain Scale	1	2	3	4	5

Next Appointment :

Follow Up Notes:

Doctor Visit Log

Date		Time:
Doctor		
Hospital / Clinic		
Phone No.		

Reasons For The Visit	Questions To Ask
Symptoms	Prescription / Tests

Pain Scale	1	2	3	4	5

Next Appointment :

Follow Up Notes:

Doctor Visit Log

Date		Time:
Doctor		
Hospital / Clinic		
Phone No.		

Reasons For The Visit	Questions To Ask
Symptoms	Prescription / Tests

Pain Scale	1	2	3	4	5

Next Appointment :

Follow Up Notes:

Doctor Visit Log

Date		Time:
Doctor		
Hospital / Clinic		
Phone No.		

Reasons For The Visit	Questions To Ask
Symptoms	Prescription / Tests

Pain Scale	1	2	3	4	5

Next Appointment :

Follow Up Notes:

Doctor Visit Log

Date		Time:
Doctor		
Hospital / Clinic		
Phone No.		

Reasons For The Visit	Questions To Ask
Symptoms	Prescription / Tests

Pain Scale	1	2	3	4	5

Next Appointment :

Follow Up Notes:

Doctor Visit Log

Date		Time:
Doctor		
Hospital / Clinic		
Phone No.		

Reasons For The Visit	Questions To Ask
Symptoms	**Prescription / Tests**

Pain Scale	1	2	3	4	5

Next Appointment :

Follow Up Notes:

Doctor Visit Log

Date		Time:
Doctor		
Hospital / Clinic		
Phone No.		

Reasons For The Visit	Questions To Ask
Symptoms	Prescription / Tests

Pain Scale	1	2	3	4	5

Next Appointment :

Follow Up Notes:

Doctor Visit Log

Date		Time:
Doctor		
Hospital / Clinic		
Phone No.		

Reasons For The Visit	Questions To Ask
Symptoms	Prescription / Tests

Pain Scale	1	2	3	4	5

Next Appointment :

Follow Up Notes:

Doctor Visit Log

Date		Time:
Doctor		
Hospital / Clinic		
Phone No.		

Reasons For The Visit	Questions To Ask
Symptoms	Prescription / Tests

Pain Scale	1	2	3	4	5

Next Appointment :

Follow Up Notes:

Doctor Visit Log

Date		Time:
Doctor		
Hospital / Clinic		
Phone No.		

Reasons For The Visit	Questions To Ask
Symptoms	Prescription / Tests

Pain Scale	1	2	3	4	5

Next Appointment :

Follow Up Notes:

Doctor Visit Log

Date		Time:
Doctor		
Hospital / Clinic		
Phone No.		

Reasons For The Visit	Questions To Ask
Symptoms	Prescription / Tests

Pain Scale	1	2	3	4	5

Next Appointment :

Follow Up Notes:

Doctor Visit Log

Date		Time:
Doctor		
Hospital / Clinic		
Phone No.		

Reasons For The Visit	Questions To Ask
Symptoms	**Prescription / Tests**

Pain Scale	1	2	3	4	5

Next Appointment :

Follow Up Notes:

Doctor Visit Log

Date		Time:
Doctor		
Hospital / Clinic		
Phone No.		

Reasons For The Visit	Questions To Ask
Symptoms	**Prescription / Tests**

Pain Scale	1	2	3	4	5

Next Appointment :

Follow Up Notes:

Doctor Visit Log

Date		Time:
Doctor		
Hospital / Clinic		
Phone No.		

Reasons For The Visit	Questions To Ask
Symptoms	**Prescription / Tests**

Pain Scale	1	2	3	4	5

Next Appointment :

Follow Up Notes:

Doctor Visit Log

Date		Time:
Doctor		
Hospital / Clinic		
Phone No.		

Reasons For The Visit	Questions To Ask
Symptoms	Prescription / Tests

Pain Scale	1	2	3	4	5

Next Appointment :

Follow Up Notes:

Doctor Visit Log

Date		Time:
Doctor		
Hospital / Clinic		
Phone No.		

Reasons For The Visit	Questions To Ask
Symptoms	Prescription / Tests

Pain Scale	1	2	3	4	5

Next Appointment :

Follow Up Notes:

Doctor Visit Log

Date		Time:
Doctor		
Hospital / Clinic		
Phone No.		

Reasons For The Visit	Questions To Ask
Symptoms	Prescription / Tests

Pain Scale	1	2	3	4	5

Next Appointment :

Follow Up Notes:

Doctor Visit Log

Date		Time:
Doctor		
Hospital / Clinic		
Phone No.		

Reasons For The Visit	Questions To Ask
Symptoms	Prescription / Tests

Pain Scale	1	2	3	4	5

Next Appointment :

Follow Up Notes:

Doctor Visit Log

Date		Time:
Doctor		
Hospital / Clinic		
Phone No.		

Reasons For The Visit	Questions To Ask
Symptoms	Prescription / Tests

Pain Scale	1	2	3	4	5

Next Appointment :

Follow Up Notes:

Doctor Visit Log

Date		Time:
Doctor		
Hospital / Clinic		
Phone No.		

Reasons For The Visit	Questions To Ask
Symptoms	**Prescription / Tests**

Pain Scale	1	2	3	4	5

Next Appointment :

Follow Up Notes:

Doctor Visit Log

Date		Time:
Doctor		
Hospital / Clinic		
Phone No.		

Reasons For The Visit	Questions To Ask
Symptoms	Prescription / Tests

Pain Scale	1	2	3	4	5

Next Appointment :

Follow Up Notes:

Doctor Visit Log

Date		Time:
Doctor		
Hospital / Clinic		
Phone No.		

Reasons For The Visit	Questions To Ask
Symptoms	Prescription / Tests

Pain Scale	1	2	3	4	5

Next Appointment :

Follow Up Notes:

Doctor Visit Log

Date		Time:
Doctor		
Hospital / Clinic		
Phone No.		

Reasons For The Visit	Questions To Ask
Symptoms	**Prescription / Tests**

Pain Scale	1	2	3	4	5

Next Appointment :

Follow Up Notes:

Doctor Visit Log

Date		Time:
Doctor		
Hospital / Clinic		
Phone No.		

Reasons For The Visit	Questions To Ask
Symptoms	Prescription / Tests

Pain Scale	1	2	3	4	5

Next Appointment :

Follow Up Notes:

Doctor Visit Log

Date		Time:
Doctor		
Hospital / Clinic		
Phone No.		

Reasons For The Visit	Questions To Ask
Symptoms	**Prescription / Tests**

Pain Scale	1	2	3	4	5

Next Appointment :

Follow Up Notes:

Doctor Visit Log

Date		Time:
Doctor		
Hospital / Clinic		
Phone No.		

Reasons For The Visit	Questions To Ask
Symptoms	Prescription / Tests

Pain Scale	1	2	3	4	5

Next Appointment :

Follow Up Notes:

Doctor Visit Log

Date		Time:
Doctor		
Hospital / Clinic		
Phone No.		

Reasons For The Visit	Questions To Ask
Symptoms	Prescription / Tests

Pain Scale	1	2	3	4	5

Next Appointment :

Follow Up Notes:

Doctor Visit Log

Date		Time:
Doctor		
Hospital / Clinic		
Phone No.		

Reasons For The Visit	Questions To Ask
Symptoms	Prescription / Tests

Pain Scale	1	2	3	4	5

Next Appointment :

Follow Up Notes:

Doctor Visit Log

Date		Time:
Doctor		
Hospital / Clinic		
Phone No.		

Reasons For The Visit	Questions To Ask
Symptoms	Prescription / Tests

Pain Scale	1	2	3	4	5

Next Appointment :

Follow Up Notes:

Doctor Visit Log

Date		Time:
Doctor		
Hospital / Clinic		
Phone No.		

Reasons For The Visit	Questions To Ask
Symptoms	**Prescription / Tests**

Pain Scale	1	2	3	4	5

Next Appointment :

Follow Up Notes:

Doctor Visit Log

Date		Time:
Doctor		
Hospital / Clinic		
Phone No.		

Reasons For The Visit	Questions To Ask
Symptoms	Prescription / Tests

Pain Scale	1	2	3	4	5

Next Appointment :

Follow Up Notes:

Doctor Visit Log

Date		Time:
Doctor		
Hospital / Clinic		
Phone No.		

Reasons For The Visit	Questions To Ask
Symptoms	Prescription / Tests

Pain Scale	1	2	3	4	5

Next Appointment :

Follow Up Notes:

Doctor Visit Log

Date		Time:
Doctor		
Hospital / Clinic		
Phone No.		

Reasons For The Visit	Questions To Ask
Symptoms	**Prescription / Tests**

Pain Scale	1	2	3	4	5

Next Appointment :

Follow Up Notes:

Doctor Visit Log

Date		Time:
Doctor		
Hospital / Clinic		
Phone No.		

Reasons For The Visit	Questions To Ask
Symptoms	Prescription / Tests

Pain Scale	1	2	3	4	5

Next Appointment :

Follow Up Notes:

Doctor Visit Log

Date		Time:
Doctor		
Hospital / Clinic		
Phone No.		

Reasons For The Visit	Questions To Ask
Symptoms	**Prescription / Tests**

Pain Scale	1	2	3	4	5

Next Appointment :

Follow Up Notes:

Doctor Visit Log

Date		Time:
Doctor		
Hospital / Clinic		
Phone No.		

Reasons For The Visit	Questions To Ask
Symptoms	Prescription / Tests

Pain Scale	1	2	3	4	5

Next Appointment :

Follow Up Notes:

Doctor Visit Log

Date		Time:
Doctor		
Hospital / Clinic		
Phone No.		

Reasons For The Visit	Questions To Ask
Symptoms	Prescription / Tests

Pain Scale	1	2	3	4	5

Next Appointment :

Follow Up Notes:

Doctor Visit Log

Date		Time:
Doctor		
Hospital / Clinic		
Phone No.		

Reasons For The Visit	Questions To Ask
Symptoms	Prescription / Tests

Pain Scale	1	2	3	4	5

Next Appointment :

Follow Up Notes:

Doctor Visit Log

Date		Time:
Doctor		
Hospital / Clinic		
Phone No.		

Reasons For The Visit	Questions To Ask
Symptoms	Prescription / Tests

Pain Scale	1	2	3	4	5

Next Appointment :

Follow Up Notes:

Doctor Visit Log

Date		Time:
Doctor		
Hospital / Clinic		
Phone No.		

Reasons For The Visit	Questions To Ask
Symptoms	**Prescription / Tests**

Pain Scale	1	2	3	4	5

Next Appointment :

Follow Up Notes:

Doctor Visit Log

Date		Time:
Doctor		
Hospital / Clinic		
Phone No.		

Reasons For The Visit	Questions To Ask
Symptoms	**Prescription / Tests**

Pain Scale	1	2	3	4	5

Next Appointment :

Follow Up Notes:

Doctor Visit Log

Date		Time:
Doctor		
Hospital / Clinic		
Phone No.		

Reasons For The Visit	Questions To Ask
Symptoms	Prescription / Tests

Pain Scale	1	2	3	4	5

Next Appointment :

Follow Up Notes:

Doctor Visit Log

Date		Time:
Doctor		
Hospital / Clinic		
Phone No.		

Reasons For The Visit	Questions To Ask
Symptoms	Prescription / Tests

Pain Scale	1	2	3	4	5

Next Appointment :

Follow Up Notes:

Doctor Visit Log

Date		Time:
Doctor		
Hospital / Clinic		
Phone No.		

Reasons For The Visit	Questions To Ask
Symptoms	Prescription / Tests

Pain Scale	1	2	3	4	5

Next Appointment :

Follow Up Notes:

Doctor Visit Log

Date		Time:
Doctor		
Hospital / Clinic		
Phone No.		

Reasons For The Visit	Questions To Ask
Symptoms	Prescription / Tests

Pain Scale	1	2	3	4	5

Next Appointment :

Follow Up Notes:

Doctor Visit Log

Date		Time:
Doctor		
Hospital / Clinic		
Phone No.		

Reasons For The Visit	Questions To Ask
Symptoms	Prescription / Tests

Pain Scale	1	2	3	4	5

Next Appointment :

Follow Up Notes:

Doctor Visit Log

Date		Time:
Doctor		
Hospital / Clinic		
Phone No.		

Reasons For The Visit	Questions To Ask
Symptoms	Prescription / Tests

Pain Scale	1	2	3	4	5

Next Appointment :

Follow Up Notes:

Doctor Visit Log

Date		Time:
Doctor		
Hospital / Clinic		
Phone No.		

Reasons For The Visit	Questions To Ask
Symptoms	Prescription / Tests

Pain Scale	1	2	3	4	5

Next Appointment :

Follow Up Notes:

Doctor Visit Log

Date		Time:
Doctor		
Hospital / Clinic		
Phone No.		

Reasons For The Visit	Questions To Ask
Symptoms	**Prescription / Tests**

Pain Scale	1	2	3	4	5

Next Appointment :

Follow Up Notes:

Doctor Visit Log

Date		Time:
Doctor		
Hospital / Clinic		
Phone No.		

Reasons For The Visit	Questions To Ask
Symptoms	Prescription / Tests

Pain Scale	1	2	3	4	5

Next Appointment :

Follow Up Notes:

Doctor Visit Log

Date		Time:
Doctor		
Hospital / Clinic		
Phone No.		

Reasons For The Visit	Questions To Ask
Symptoms	Prescription / Tests

Pain Scale	1	2	3	4	5

Next Appointment :

Follow Up Notes:

Doctor Visit Log

Date		Time:
Doctor		
Hospital / Clinic		
Phone No.		

Reasons For The Visit	Questions To Ask
Symptoms	Prescription / Tests

Pain Scale	1	2	3	4	5

Next Appointment :

Follow Up Notes:

Doctor Visit Log

Date		Time:
Doctor		
Hospital / Clinic		
Phone No.		

Reasons For The Visit	Questions To Ask
Symptoms	Prescription / Tests

Pain Scale	1	2	3	4	5

Next Appointment :

Follow Up Notes:

Doctor Visit Log

Date		Time:
Doctor		
Hospital / Clinic		
Phone No.		

Reasons For The Visit	Questions To Ask
Symptoms	Prescription / Tests

Pain Scale	1	2	3	4	5

Next Appointment :

Follow Up Notes:

Doctor Visit Log

Date		Time:
Doctor		
Hospital / Clinic		
Phone No.		

Reasons For The Visit	Questions To Ask
Symptoms	Prescription / Tests

Pain Scale	1	2	3	4	5

Next Appointment :

Follow Up Notes:

Doctor Visit Log

Date		Time:
Doctor		
Hospital / Clinic		
Phone No.		

Reasons For The Visit	Questions To Ask
Symptoms	**Prescription / Tests**

Pain Scale	1	2	3	4	5

Next Appointment :

Follow Up Notes:

Doctor Visit Log

Date		Time:
Doctor		
Hospital / Clinic		
Phone No.		

Reasons For The Visit	Questions To Ask
Symptoms	**Prescription / Tests**

Pain Scale	1	2	3	4	5

Next Appointment :

Follow Up Notes:

Doctor Visit Log

Date		Time:
Doctor		
Hospital / Clinic		
Phone No.		

Reasons For The Visit	Questions To Ask
Symptoms	**Prescription / Tests**

Pain Scale	1	2	3	4	5

Next Appointment :

Follow Up Notes:

Doctor Visit Log

Date		Time:
Doctor		
Hospital / Clinic		
Phone No.		

Reasons For The Visit	Questions To Ask
Symptoms	Prescription / Tests

Pain Scale	1	2	3	4	5

Next Appointment :

Follow Up Notes:

Doctor Visit Log

Date		Time:
Doctor		
Hospital / Clinic		
Phone No.		

Reasons For The Visit	Questions To Ask
Symptoms	Prescription / Tests

Pain Scale	1	2	3	4	5

Next Appointment :

Follow Up Notes:

Doctor Visit Log

Date		Time:
Doctor		
Hospital / Clinic		
Phone No.		

Reasons For The Visit	Questions To Ask
Symptoms	Prescription / Tests

Pain Scale	1	2	3	4	5

Next Appointment :

Follow Up Notes:

Doctor Visit Log

Date		Time:
Doctor		
Hospital / Clinic		
Phone No.		

Reasons For The Visit	Questions To Ask
Symptoms	Prescription / Tests

Pain Scale	1	2	3	4	5

Next Appointment :

Follow Up Notes:

Doctor Visit Log

Date		Time:
Doctor		
Hospital / Clinic		
Phone No.		

Reasons For The Visit	Questions To Ask
Symptoms	Prescription / Tests

Pain Scale	1	2	3	4	5

Next Appointment :

Follow Up Notes:

Doctor Visit Log

Date		Time:
Doctor		
Hospital / Clinic		
Phone No.		

Reasons For The Visit	Questions To Ask
Symptoms	Prescription / Tests

Pain Scale	1	2	3	4	5

Next Appointment :

Follow Up Notes:

Doctor Visit Log

Date		Time:
Doctor		
Hospital / Clinic		
Phone No.		

Reasons For The Visit	Questions To Ask
Symptoms	Prescription / Tests

Pain Scale	1	2	3	4	5

Next Appointment :

Follow Up Notes:

Doctor Visit Log

Date		Time:
Doctor		
Hospital / Clinic		
Phone No.		

Reasons For The Visit	Questions To Ask
Symptoms	Prescription / Tests

Pain Scale	1	2	3	4	5

Next Appointment :

Follow Up Notes:

Doctor Visit Log

Date		Time:
Doctor		
Hospital / Clinic		
Phone No.		

Reasons For The Visit	Questions To Ask
Symptoms	Prescription / Tests

Pain Scale	1	2	3	4	5

Next Appointment :

Follow Up Notes:

Doctor Visit Log

Date		Time:
Doctor		
Hospital / Clinic		
Phone No.		

Reasons For The Visit	Questions To Ask
Symptoms	**Prescription / Tests**

Pain Scale	1	2	3	4	5

Next Appointment :

Follow Up Notes:

Doctor Visit Log

Date		Time:
Doctor		
Hospital / Clinic		
Phone No.		

Reasons For The Visit	Questions To Ask
Symptoms	**Prescription / Tests**

Pain Scale	1	2	3	4	5

Next Appointment :

Follow Up Notes:

Doctor Visit Log

Date		Time:
Doctor		
Hospital / Clinic		
Phone No.		

Reasons For The Visit	Questions To Ask
Symptoms	Prescription / Tests

Pain Scale	1	2	3	4	5

Next Appointment :

Follow Up Notes:

Doctor Visit Log

Date		Time:
Doctor		
Hospital / Clinic		
Phone No.		

Reasons For The Visit	Questions To Ask
Symptoms	**Prescription / Tests**

Pain Scale	1	2	3	4	5

Next Appointment :

Follow Up Notes:

Doctor Visit Log

Date		Time:
Doctor		
Hospital / Clinic		
Phone No.		

Reasons For The Visit	Questions To Ask
Symptoms	Prescription / Tests

Pain Scale	1	2	3	4	5

Next Appointment :

Follow Up Notes:

Doctor Visit Log

Date		Time:
Doctor		
Hospital / Clinic		
Phone No.		

Reasons For The Visit	Questions To Ask
Symptoms	Prescription / Tests

Pain Scale	1	2	3	4	5

Next Appointment :

Follow Up Notes:

Doctor Visit Log

Date		Time:
Doctor		
Hospital / Clinic		
Phone No.		

Reasons For The Visit	Questions To Ask
Symptoms	Prescription / Tests

Pain Scale	1	2	3	4	5

Next Appointment :

Follow Up Notes:

Doctor Visit Log

Date		Time:
Doctor		
Hospital / Clinic		
Phone No.		

Reasons For The Visit	Questions To Ask
Symptoms	**Prescription / Tests**

Pain Scale	1	2	3	4	5

Next Appointment :

Follow Up Notes:

Doctor Visit Log

Date		Time:
Doctor		
Hospital / Clinic		
Phone No.		

Reasons For The Visit	Questions To Ask
Symptoms	**Prescription / Tests**

Pain Scale	1	2	3	4	5

Next Appointment :

Follow Up Notes:

Doctor Visit Log

Date		Time:
Doctor		
Hospital / Clinic		
Phone No.		

Reasons For The Visit	Questions To Ask
Symptoms	Prescription / Tests

Pain Scale	1	2	3	4	5

Next Appointment :

Follow Up Notes:

Doctor Visit Log

Date		Time:
Doctor		
Hospital / Clinic		
Phone No.		

Reasons For The Visit	Questions To Ask
Symptoms	**Prescription / Tests**

Pain Scale	1	2	3	4	5

Next Appointment :

Follow Up Notes:

Doctor Visit Log

Date		Time:
Doctor		
Hospital / Clinic		
Phone No.		

Reasons For The Visit	Questions To Ask
Symptoms	Prescription / Tests

Pain Scale	1	2	3	4	5

Next Appointment :

Follow Up Notes:

Doctor Visit Log

Date		Time:
Doctor		
Hospital / Clinic		
Phone No.		

Reasons For The Visit	Questions To Ask
Symptoms	Prescription / Tests

Pain Scale	1	2	3	4	5

Next Appointment :

Follow Up Notes:

Doctor Visit Log

Date		Time:
Doctor		
Hospital / Clinic		
Phone No.		

Reasons For The Visit	Questions To Ask
Symptoms	Prescription / Tests

Pain Scale	1	2	3	4	5

Next Appointment :

Follow Up Notes:

Doctor Visit Log

Date		Time:
Doctor		
Hospital / Clinic		
Phone No.		

Reasons For The Visit	Questions To Ask
Symptoms	Prescription / Tests

Pain Scale	1	2	3	4	5

Next Appointment :

Follow Up Notes:

Doctor Visit Log

Date		Time:
Doctor		
Hospital / Clinic		
Phone No.		

Reasons For The Visit	Questions To Ask
Symptoms	Prescription / Tests

Pain Scale	1	2	3	4	5

Next Appointment :

Follow Up Notes:

Doctor Visit Log

Date		Time:
Doctor		
Hospital / Clinic		
Phone No.		

Reasons For The Visit	Questions To Ask
Symptoms	**Prescription / Tests**

Pain Scale	1	2	3	4	5

Next Appointment :

Follow Up Notes:

Doctor Visit Log

Date		Time:
Doctor		
Hospital / Clinic		
Phone No.		

Reasons For The Visit	Questions To Ask
Symptoms	**Prescription / Tests**

Pain Scale	1	2	3	4	5

Next Appointment :

Follow Up Notes:

Doctor Visit Log

Date		Time:
Doctor		
Hospital / Clinic		
Phone No.		

Reasons For The Visit	Questions To Ask
Symptoms	Prescription / Tests

Pain Scale	1	2	3	4	5

Next Appointment :

Follow Up Notes:

Doctor Visit Log

Date		Time:
Doctor		
Hospital / Clinic		
Phone No.		

Reasons For The Visit	Questions To Ask
Symptoms	**Prescription / Tests**

Pain Scale	1	2	3	4	5

Next Appointment :

Follow Up Notes:

Doctor Visit Log

Date		Time:
Doctor		
Hospital / Clinic		
Phone No.		

Reasons For The Visit	Questions To Ask
Symptoms	**Prescription / Tests**

Pain Scale	1	2	3	4	5

Next Appointment :

Follow Up Notes:

Doctor Visit Log

Date		Time:
Doctor		
Hospital / Clinic		
Phone No.		

Reasons For The Visit	Questions To Ask
Symptoms	**Prescription / Tests**

Pain Scale	1	2	3	4	5

Next Appointment :

Follow Up Notes:

Made in the USA
Monee, IL
07 July 2026